Lukas Falvey

DIET EXPRESS

...about diets and weight loss

TABLE OF CONTENTS

CHAPTER ONE

INTRODUCTION

The term diet comes from the ancient Greek δίαιτα díaita and was originally used in the sense of "lifestyle" / "way of life". The dietetics deals still scientifically with the "right" diet and lifestyle. In German-speaking countries, the term refers to certain diets and diets that are intended either to gain or lose weight or to treat diseases. Colloquially, the term in Germany is often equated with a reduction diet (Reduktionsdiät) for weight loss. It is therefore a synonym for the slimming diet.

DIET FORMS

Since Hippocrates, a special diet for humans has been called a diet, in which a special selection of foods is consumed over the long term or permanently. The diet is either a short-term change in diet for weight reduction (e.g. in the case of obesity), in some cases also for weight gain (e.g. in the case of anorexia) or a longer-term or permanent change in diet to support the treatment of an illness (e.g. B. in celiac disease, lactose intolerance, fructose intolerance).

Fasting, on the other hand, means temporarily avoiding food for religious reasons (Ramadan in Islam, pre-Easter fasting in the Christian church) or health reasons (therapeutic fasting). Every form of diet, whether it is used for weight reduction or for supporting disease treatment, is based on a decrease or increase in the relative proportion of one food component (carbohydrates, fats, proteins, vitamins, minerals and preservatives) compared to the others and / or a decrease or increase in the amount consumed Total amount of energy and, if applicable, a balanced change in fluid intake.

Cognitive behavior therapy, which psychologists use in clinics to treat obesity, takes a more holistic approach. With this method, dysfunctional behavior and eating habits are identified and retrained. If you are very overweight and have eating disorders, it is considered to be the most sensible long-term method for weight loss.

REDUCTION DIETS

Example of lunch with a reduced diet

A weight loss diet aims to reduce body weight. There are numerous reduction diets, some of which differ considerably in their methods. Only a few diet forms have been scientifically verified. The development and propagation of the reduction diets is not only subject to changes in scientific knowledge, but also to fashions and world views. Some forms of diet are even considered hazardous to health in medicine. There are numerous diets with different conceptions. These are called, for example, low-carb, low-fat, food combining or glyx diet. In a weight loss diet, reducing your carbohydrate intake is just as effective as reducing your fat intake.

DISEASE TREATMENT DIETS

Diets are used as a single measure or in addition to medicinal and possibly surgical therapy for the treatment of diseases. Nutritional medicine deals with the development of effective nutritional strategies. Until the 1980s, almost every disease had its own diet. Nowadays, for most diseases, as well as for the general population, a possibly modified, lacto-vegetarian whole food diet in connection with physical activity is recommended. Particularly in the treatment of diabetes, there has been a paradigm shift since the 1990s, which led away from a very strictly regulated diet to an almost complete release of the dietary recommendations (" energy-reduced mixed diet ").

How does exercise affect a diet?

- o **The goal:** the exercise increases the daily requirement of calories. Furthermore, depending on the type of exercise or training, the metabolism increases. In short: The movement ensures a higher energy consumption and thus leads to a faster achievement of the goal.

- o **Stress reduction:** In addition to normal everyday life, a diet can mean stress because you have to deal more with nutrition and do without a lot. This stress is relieved through exercise, provided you choose a sport that you enjoy.

- **Endorphins:** During exercise, happiness hormones (= endorphins) are released. These are of course also distributed when consuming sweets. But no, forget it, they are no longer allowed! So to still get this great feeling, you just have to "just" move.

- **More motivation:** You started a diet because you have a specific goal, let's say lose 20kg. In the beginning it goes quite well, you lose weight quickly and you are motivated. But after a while, the weight loss stagnates. At the latest, at the very latest now, sport must be integrated into your everyday life, because the aforementioned aspects come into play and you will achieve your goal.

CHAPTER TWO

WEIGHT REDUCTION

Types of weight loss

The (human) body can lose weight through loss of water, breakdown of reserve substances such as glycogen or body fat, muscle mass, minerals, bone loss and loss of body parts and hair. By breathing is only minimal weight loss (exhaled CO_2 - molecules are slightly heavier than O_2 molecules).

- **Loss of water**

The water content of the human body can be between 45 and 70%, depending on your personal constitution. More obese people carry proportionally less water with them because fat tissue contains less water than muscle tissue, for example. Apart from dehydration (desiccosis due to decreased fluid intake or insufficient fluid intake, see dehydration), the short-term decrease in body water can lead to a supposedly rapid weight loss.

Phosphates are used in food processing to provide preparations (for example ham, sausage, processed cheese) with more water (for better process ability, "juicier" appearance or food fraud so that water is sold at sausage price). From this, unproven hypotheses were derived that phosphates supplied with food would also bind water in the body.

- **Breakdown of glycogen**

In a person weighing 80 kg, around two to two and a half kilograms of hydrous glycogen are stored. This glycogen store in muscles and liver is available to endurance athletes or is primarily reduced during a diet. As a polysaccharide, like starch, glycogen is highly hygroscopic and is therefore stored in the cells with the help of water. The often rapid weight loss in the first few days of low-carb diets can be explained by the loss of this water. Consistent with this, the continuation of the habitual eating behavior leads to the replenishment of the glycogen stores in the body and an extremely rapid increase in weight of up to 2-3 kg due to the storage of water.

- **Targeted weight reduction to reduce excess weight**

Targeted weight reduction is especially necessary in the case of obesity, which often occurs in industrialized countries, where only a few people do hard physical work and where food is in abundance. If you are very overweight (obese), measures of bariatric surgery can also be used. The goal is to achieve the "ideal weight" or at least to reduce excess weight.

The following positive effects are expected:

- Fewer diseases ("better health") and at the same time higher life expectancy
- To be able to perform and to withstand stress (increased fitness)
- More zest for life
- Slimmer appearance

- **Weight loss as a result of diseases and disorders**

Physical, mental, and behavioral (eating disorder) disorders can result in weight loss. Misguided self-awareness can lead to underweight.

CHAPTER THREE

INTERMITTENT FASTING

Intermittent fasting - also called interval fasting - alternates phases of not eating with phases of normal food intake. Instead of eating for a longer period of several days and thus restricting yourself considerably, fasting is done every hour by the hour. The idea behind it: manageable periods make it easier to do without and the probability of the yo-yo effect is less. There is less of a nagging feeling of hunger - often a reason for food cravings that completely negate the success of the diet. It is also believed that the body "digests" such short-term food restrictions better than long-term fasting. The 16:8 methods are only one solution, there are other forms of interval fasting. This includes, for example, the 5:2 methods: here you can eat normally on five days and fast on two.

Intermittent fasting is followed by periods of normal nutrition after periods without food intake. The rhythm between normal food intake and fasting is constant and a 24-hour change in most laboratory tests. This means that a phase of 24 hours of fasting is followed by a phase of 24 hours of normal nutrition. During the fasting period, solid food was usually completely dispensed with in the experiments and liquid intake only took the form of water. This form of nutrition is described in the Anglo-Saxon literature every other day diet (EOD) or alternate day fasting (ADF) called.

Another version of interval fasting is that the switch between fasting and eating periods takes place within a day. The 16:8 methods are often used. An 8-hour phase of food intake only begins after a 16-hour food waiting period. Taking into account the night's rest and the absence of breakfast or dinner, this procedure can be integrated into the daily routine without major changes, since the diet does not have to be changed. During the fasting block, water and unsweetened tea or coffee are allowed. In the case of daily rhythm interval fasting, variants with even longer food breaks (e.g. 18:6 or 20:4) are propagated.

Intermittent fasting leads to similar physiological and metabolic changes in humans as a continuous calorie restriction. A major difference, however, is that significantly higher plasma concentrations of keto bodies can be detected in intermittent fasting. It is believed that the pattern of intermittent fasting more closely resembles that of humans before the beginning of agriculture and animal husbandry than the eating rhythms of modern times and that the human body is still adapted to this.

Broader clinical experience comes from countries with a predominantly Muslim population in which Ramadan is celebrated annually. The observed metabolic improvements in healthy people are very small. Other studies describe an increase in unfavorable LDL cholesterol and a decrease in good HDL cholesterol, especially in healthy men. In overweight people who practice Ramadan, the improved body composition returns to the initial state after a few weeks.

HEALTH BENEFITS OF INTERMITTENT FASTING

The advantages which brings the intermittent fasting with them are varied and reach every corner of the body: the fat burning is increased inflammatory processes are inhibited, improve cholesterol levels in the blood itself, in the brain new nerve cells are overproduced. This reduces age-related risk factors, you lose weight more easily and it is also reasonable to assume that the effects of such a nutritional behavior prolong life. Intermittent fasting is an ormetic stimulus: it means that if it is dosed in the correct way it produces a reparative and reinforcing response by the body, as happens in the case of physical training. This stimulus is triggered by the caloric deficit and induces numerous changes: the body adapts its hormonal levels, the cells initiate the repair and autophagy processes towards the damaged ones and the gene expression is modulated, as well as the insulin response.

In our modern world, people often like to consume several times a day unconsciously and almost as a snack, and thus always add calories to the body. For a long time, not eating anything means subjectively perceived stress for many people. And it is actually a kind of stress for the body, because our cells are irritated or stressed to a small extent. And this is exactly what can do us good: Similar to sport, this mild stress trains the cells and makes our body more resistant to more severe stress factors such as diseases (principle of hormesis). In fact, a reduced meal frequency leads to a reduction in risk factors for Alzheimer's and diabetes, Cardiovascular diseases and many other diseases.

The benefits of intermittent fasting on your health:

- Improvement of the digestive tract
- Regulation of blood sugar levels
- Increased fat burning and losing weight
- Easier entry into ketosis and increased mental performance
- Faster regeneration of nerve cells

Advantages:

- Gentle form of weight loss without too much sacrifice
- Intermittent fasting can be built into everyday life
- Only fat, no muscle mass is lost
- A good method against the yo-yo effect
- Food cravings are reduced to a minimum
- No feelings of weakness as normal food intake

Disadvantage:

- Only a limited weight loss effect without a real reduction in energy supply
- Weight reductions are rather slow - but sustainable
- 16 hours without food cause problems for some people
- Depending on the daily schedule and working hours, not always easy to implement.

WHY CALORIES LOSS COUNTS

A calorie is a unit of measurement that indicates the energy contained in food and is reported in kilocalories (kcal) or kilojoule (kJ). This is usually the first information provided on the label of the product purchased (before the content of carbohydrates, proteins, fats, salt, etc.). It is therefore a physical unit of measurement of energy, work and heat. This number represents the amount of heat required to raise the temperature of 1 gram of water (14.5 to 15.5 ° C) by 1°C under normal atmospheric pressure. One kilocalorie is approximately 4.18 kilojoule. It is this energy contained in the food that our body will need to ensure all the vital functions.

The basic principle of weight loss is obviously to burn more calories than you consume, and therefore have a negative energy balance at the end of the day. But not much more! If you suddenly adopt a draconian diet, i.e. very low in calories over a long period of time, your body will come to rest and go into "economy" mode to keep it functioning. It will therefore use each calorie ingested to its maximum. The consequence: as soon as you start to eat normally, you will regain weight because the body will want to store up in anticipation of a new period of restriction.

How is the basal metabolic rate calculated?

The simplest method is the following rule of thumb: basal metabolic rate = body weight (kg) x 24 hours. Example for a person weighing 70 kg: 70 x 24 = 1680 kcal basal metabolic rate per day.

How to count calories according to body weight?

Depending on the age, the basal metabolic rate of an 80 kg man amounts to 2200 to 2500 calories per day. If he does an office job, there will be more than 3000, with regular exercise the effective total turnover can quickly reach 3500 kilocalories or even more. The lower metabolic rate is necessary in old age because of the slightly reduced metabolism. Men have the advantage over women that they consume significantly more calories when at rest. This results from the different structure of the body tissue of the sexes. Men have less fat, but more muscle. As is well known, they consume significantly more energy than fat. Furthermore, the muscles of men are equipped with beta receptors, which additionally boost the body's own power plant.

In women, too, calorie requirements decrease with age. Most people notice that they gain significantly faster during and after menopause or have problems getting rid of the extra pounds. The basal metabolism of a 60-year-old is 1700 kilocalories, while a 20-year-old woman needs 2000 calories a day. Exercise also has an impact on calorie requirements. Half an hour burns between 200 and 400 kilocalories. It is indispensable for an office job if the weight is to be kept or reduced. Due to the higher proportion of estrogen in the blood, but also due to the artificially added hormones such as those contained in the pill, women are quicker to gain love.

In addition, a woman's body is programmed by evolution to put on fat for times of need and create enough reserves for pregnancy. In any case, the basic metabolic rate is increased by around 500 kilocalories a day during pregnancy, and even by 800 kcal during breastfeeding. Because women have less muscle than men, weight training is ideal for them. This increases the overall turnover and the so-called "after burn effect" after the training also causes further calorie loss.

What does calorie requirement mean?

Calories almost always play a role when it comes to losing weight. However, very few people know how many calories they can consume a day so that they can lose weight or avoid gaining weight. There is no one calorie requirement for everyone. Because how many calories a person can consume per day depends on gender, age and size. Factors such as regular exercise, sport and work also play a role. After all, a worker on a construction site requires significantly more energy than an employee in the office. Even so, most calories are burned at rest. 70 percent. The body needs the amount supplied for its basic metabolism.

The technical term for this is basal metabolic rate. The basal metabolic rate ensures that all vital functions are maintained. This includes breathing, heartbeat and supply to the individual organs. However, many people eat well above their daily calorie needs, which sooner or later becomes apparent as being overweight. Others reduce their calorie needs to lose weight so much that they slide into a hunger metabolism. If you know your daily needs, you can take appropriate precautions to keep the pounds from falling or to keep the weight off. Some people who are underweight need to be careful about gaining weight. It is also important for them to know the calorie needs.

COMBINING "IF" AND KETOGENIC DIET

Intermittent fasting itself already has numerous advantages and does not only focus on reducing weight. Intermittent fasting in combination with ketogenic nutrition is an absolute boost for weight loss, body fat reduction and also for the implementation of the advantages mentioned above. You get into ketosis faster because of the faster emptying of the carbohydrate stores. Basically it is not difficult to combine these two nutritional methods with each other. They even fit together very well and the effect is great because you take advantage of both forms and lose weight even faster and primarily lose body fat and hardly any muscle.

Studies show that the combination of keto and interval fasting is the nutritional form where the body fat percentage is reduced the most.

The advantages of both diets at a glance:

Benefits of a ketogenic diet:

- Fast weight loss and body fat reduction
- Increase in mental and physical performance and endurance (through more even energy supply than with carbohydrate metabolism)
- Keeps blood sugar levels steady and prevents cravings ago
- Better ability to concentrate through "ketolysis" (ability to use ketone bodies for energy)
- Balance blood pressure and lower high blood pressure
- Reversing Type 2 Diabetes
- Cure migraines
- Control of epilepsy and reduction of medication
- Better complexion, reduce inflammation and pimples
- Reduce stomach pain & nausea
- Decrease heart rate

Advantages of interval fasting:

- Fast weight loss
- Better concentration
- Less morning headache
- Less dyspnea (shortness of breath) under stress or even at rest
- Less sleep and sleep problems
- You are much more awake during the day
- Your physical performance improves
- You age more slowly
- Less cardiovascular disease
- Protection against cancer and Alzheimer's
- Recovery of genes and body cells
- Blood sugar levels improve
- Insulin resistance
- Stops type 2 diabetes
- Condition improves
- Regeneration is faster
- More power when training
- The growth of new nerve cells is encouraged
- Brain function & our memory

If you want to start combining intermittent fasting with your ketogenic diet, here are a few tips for success:

- Eat the right fat, that is what helps you burn body fat faster.
- Avoid ketogenic recipes made with low carb flours (at least at the beginning of the conversion phase). Low carb flours often still have a relatively large amount of carbohydrates, which prevent you from getting into ketosis and in the worst case can even make you fat.
- Rely on the right protein sources in keto. A common mistake is that many people eat low-fat curd cheese, chicken or crabs and therefore do not get into ketosis and gain weight.
- Check! Measure your ketone levels with Ketosis and make sure you are actually in ketosis. While fasting can really help you stay in the state of ketosis, it is still important that you take care not to overeat protein or carbohydrates.

16:8 INTERVAL FASTING GUIDE

The basis of the 16:8 interval fasting diet is the daily clearly regulated rhythm of a 16-hour meal break and 8-hour time with normal food intake. This is very different from the normal daily routine we all know. For example, it looks like this:

- Breakfast 7 a.m.
- Lunch at 12 noon
- Dinner at 7 p.m.

There are phases of several hours between the meal times. The longest is - due to sleep - the period between dinner and breakfast, 12 hours in the previous example. The other meal breaks are shorter. Often, snacks are also consumed between large meals.

16:8 interval fasting plan without breakfast

Intermittent fasting means a change in time, because there must be a 16-hour fast. Many find it particularly easy to forego breakfast or to put it behind. It can look like this:

- Lunch at 12 noon
- Afternoon snack 4 p.m.
- Dinner at 8 p.m.

In this case there is exactly 16 hours of fasting between lunch and dinner.

16:8 interval fasting plan without dinner

In the same way, you can also have a good breakfast and have a nice meal in the afternoon and skip dinner. An example would be the following interval fasting plan:

- Breakfast 8 a.m.
- Lunch at 12 noon
- Afternoon snack 4 p.m.

Here, too, there is a 16-hour interval between afternoon snack and breakfast, during which you are not allowed to eat. How you best divide that up also depends on the other daily routine. In the beginning, it is difficult for some to adhere to the 16-hour meal break. To get used to it, a vegetable broth or a little unsweetened tea is allowed in between. Some start with a break of 14 hours and then gradually approach the 16 hours.

16:8 interval fasting - what and how much can you eat?

Strictly speaking, 16:8 interval fasting is not a diet. Because the food intake is actually only distributed differently in time than usual. This makes it easier to engage in this form of fasting. A diet effect often occurs due to the time limitation of food intake, but this is limited.

The reason for this is that the body changes certain metabolic processes through the 16 hours of fasting. On the one hand, the insulin level drops, which stimulates fat burning.

On the other hand, the number of human growth hormones (HGH) also increases significantly, which in turn increases fat burning. Already these changed processes lead to weight loss, even if the food intake remains largely identical. However, weight loss can be increased significantly if you adjust your food intake and make it healthier in parallel to fasting. Fasting becomes a "true" diet only when you restrict your diet, which makes sense for previously unhealthy diets. A food restriction means a reduction in calorie intake.

For whom is 16:8 fasting suitable - and for whom not?

16:8 interval fasting suits many people who want to "lose weight" without having to restrict themselves too much. Even those who only want to maintain their existing weight are well served with the method. In the 8-hour meal phase, some "sins" are even allowed without having a guilty conscience. Sporty people are also fond of interval fasting, because the sport activities can be perfectly integrated into the 16:8 rhythms - ideally during

Lent, while new energy is being refueled during meal time.

The method is not so suitable for overweight people because it does not bring enough and only slow weight loss. Interval fasting should be combined with a change in diet and a daily calorie deficit in the form of a reduction diet. Even those who find it difficult to do without food for 16 hours will find it difficult to persevere. But there are also a few health contraindications. Intermittent fasting should not be done during pregnancy and breastfeeding. Fasting is also less suitable for older people. Other contraindications are:

- Cardiovascular problems
- Low blood pressure
- Metabolic diseases
- Chronic diseases

How much do you lose in 16:8 interval fasting?

The answer to this question is: it depends on everyone and of course on the circumstances. If you start too many pounds, you have more to lose. Those who start fasting relatively lean need not lose much. Calorie intake also plays a crucial role during the meal phase. If the energy supply covers the body's energy requirements during this time, weight loss will be kept within narrow limits. Weight loss will generally be slower than with some crash diets, but success is more sustainable in many cases - for example, due to the lack of a yo-yo effect. With a clear restriction on eating, a decrease of five to ten kilograms during a six to eight-week fasting period is quite possible.

Is intermittent fasting healthy?

In a nutshell: yes. In addition to weight loss, the method is said to have many other positive effects. The 16-hour meal waiver gives the body a break in which toxins can be excreted and detoxification takes place. The liver is relieved. The body's own insulin can be processed better, so fasting has a diabetes-preventive effect. The sugar and fat metabolism is better regulated, blood pressure and cholesterol levels are more in balance.

Another positive effect compared to other diets is that no muscle mass is lost with normal food intake. As a result, the body appears firmer overall. Intermittent fasting is also said to have a positive effect or prevent ailments such as rheumatism, multiple sclerosis, chronic pain, dementia and even cancer. Here, however, scientific proof is again required in a special way. If anything, there are only findings from laboratory tests.

How long should 16:8 interval fasting take?

Basically, there is no time limit as long as the body gets what it needs. If you want, the principle of "16 hours not eating - 8 hours of normal food intake" can be maintained for a lifetime. Another question is whether you want to submit to such a strict rhythm in the long run. Intermittent fasting as a permanent solution only makes sense if you also feel comfortable with it. A real diet, in which the body receives less energy than it needs, must always be limited. The rule applies here: rather less waiver, but longer and more sustainable.

OTHER TYPES OF FASTING METHOD

Intermittent fasting differs from strict fasting in several ways. Their main difference is that intermittent fasting is, by definition, an alternation of periods of fasting and periods of food intake. Strict fasting is a fast during which no food is taken. We had already written a full article on the subject of this type of fasting. So here are the different types of intermittent fasting described in a clear and detailed way. There are six different types of intermittent fasting that can help you lose weight while improving your health. Be careful, however, to take care to follow these different diets to the letter, whatever the choice. This so that they can have an effective action and that they do not cause health problems, due to a bad practice of the latter.

1.   THE 16/8 METHOD

This type of intermittent fasting consists of alternating periods. First, there will be a meal between 8 and 10 hours. Then there will be a fasting period of 2 to 4 p.m. This includes two, three or more meals. For example: have a snack at 4 p.m. and no longer eat until breakfast the next day (between 6 a.m. and 8 a.m.). This is equivalent to a fasting period of 14 to 16 hours in total.

2.   EAT STOP EAT

In the category of different types of intermittent fasting, we also find the Eat Stop Eat. This type of fast is translated in French as "Eat-Stop-Manger". It is done by doing one to two full days of 24 hour fasting each week. For example, when the fast begins on Tuesday at noon, it must end the next day at the same time. That is to say until Wednesday at noon. Note that during periods of fasting, solid foods are not allowed. However, calorie-free drinks (water, coffee, tea, etc.) are.

3.   THE WARRIOR DIET

The Warrior Diet, translates into French as "the warrior diet". It was developed by a recognized nutrition expert. It consists of fasting during the day. During the day, the consumption of small raw vegetables and small fruits is allowed. Then you have to eat a substantial meal for 4 hours at night. This type of intermittent fasting is reminiscent of the Paleo diet where you eat mostly whole, unprocessed foods. The method may seem quite surprising, but it is also very effective.

4.   IMPROVISED MEAL SKIPS

The different types of intermittent fasting, described above, all have an established and well-defined protocol. They are each to be followed rigorously. However, it is also possible not to respect a precise method, but to carry out moments of fasting as desired. In other words, we can very well skip meals at any time of the day, of the week, of the month. For example, it is quite possible not to have breakfast in the morning for any reason whatsoever. Like not being hungry, not having time, etc.

Or do not eat one evening because cooking at that time seems complicated or you are tired.

5. JUICE FASTING

What is eaten during juice fasting?

Fasting can last from one to eight days; during this time, those who are willing to diet only consume liquid food. He drinks about three liters a day - especially water and herbal teas as well as fruit juice and vegetable broth. One or more relief days with rice or raw food precede the actual fasting phase.

What is promised in juice fasting?

Juice fasting is seen by its followers as a holistic concept of self-awareness with physical and psychological effects. It should help to change habits and "detoxify" the body, "purify". Mostly, however, juice fasting is only used for slimming down.

What can this interval fasting method really do?

Juices and broth hardly provide any energy. Therefore, there is a reduction of three to six kilos per week. As with all radical approaches, a lot of water is lost. After Lent it is quickly replenished; the weight then often rises above the initial value. Purification has not been scientifically proven.

The conclusion: conditionally recommendable

Positive: With good advice or in a professionally guided group, fasting can become a positive, holistic experience. Healthy people can fast up to eight days on their own responsibility without hesitation.

Negative: Fasting does not make you slim in the long run: the actual changeover has yet to be managed. In addition, the protein deficiency threatens muscle breakdown - and the yo-yo effect.

6.   Whole days fast according to the 5:2 method

Eat what you really want on 5 days - and quick on 2 days, allowing a small quantity of food. Women are able to consume as much as 500 kcal, men as much as 600 kcal, for instance in the form of veggies, soup or fruits. So you are able to make the fasting days rather pleasant. The selection of fasting days can also be arbitrary, they must only stop being consecutive. So you are able to, for instance, take part in a birthday celebration party inside a relaxed manner or even go out to eat. It's essential to consume enough, but usually calorie free, preferably teas and water.

Plus points: The 5:2 diet is ideal for daily use and versatile. The fasting days could be kept up well, since you do not have to do without entirely. After the diet stage, you switch to just 1 day of fasting and will maintain your fat well.

Caution: Not ideal for kids, competitive athletes, pregnant women, individuals with an eating disorder and also underweight. If you've diabetes or other chronic illnesses, ask the doctor of yours.

Suitable for: People who find calorie counting too complex, but think it is easy never to eat. No demands for fats or carbohydrates. Regulates blood values.

Weight damage factor: 500 to 800 g each day of fasting are provided.

CHAPTER FOUR

VEGAN DIET

A well-planned vegan diet is healthy. It can prevent diseases of affluence and, when done correctly, contains all the essential nutrients in sufficient quantities. An overview of the advantages of a plant-based diet and what you should pay attention to. In the vegan diet it consists only of foods of plant origin. Based on the American Dietetic Association (ADA) in its opinion published in 2009 (one), well planned vegetarian diets are best suited for all phases of the life cycle, such as pregnancy, lactation, infancy, adolescence and childhood, and also for athletes. Because of this it's essential in order to understand this dietary option as well as to understand it.

Individuals that follow a vegetarian eating plan should pay particular attention to diet planning and create the needed dietary modifications to meet the needs of theirs. Health advice from a vegetarian nutritionist is recommended for a healthy and varied diet plan. The diet must evaluate the contribution of certain nutrients like calcium, vitamin B12, iron, vitamin D and Omega 3 fatty acids. If the diet doesn't include dairy, it is going to be needed to focus on calcium and vitamin D, and organize it including other vegetarian foods (of vegetable origin) which provide appreciable amounts of calcium and guarantee daily sun exposure. In some situations, supplementation to provide specific nutrients will be recommended, such as vitamin B12 supplementation if you follow a vegan diet.

The vegan diet or vegan diet consists of eliminating all foods of animal origin: meat, fish, crustaceans but also (unlike the vegetarian diet) eggs, dairy products and honey. It is mostly practiced for ethical, health and ecological reasons. By definition, the vegan diet is a lifestyle more than a diet.

Vegetarian diets

Vegetarian food is a dietary option that favors the consumption of foods of plant origin and the reduction or total elimination of foods of animal origin. Vegetarian diet in this way we can find different types of vegetarian diets:

Ovolocteovegetarian diet

It is a diet that eliminates meat and fish and their derivatives and includes, in addition to foods of plant origin, eggs and dairy.

Eliminate meats, fish and dairy products. The only food of animal origin in the ovovegetarian diet is eggs.

- **Prevent diseases**

Cardiovascular diseases, cancer, diabetes mellitus II and many other so-called prosperity diseases related to lifestyle are increasing significantly. As numerous studies have now shown, a vegan diet can help prevent these diseases. Vegans are less overweight, less likely to develop diabetes mellitus II, have less high blood pressure than omnivores and have lower cholesterol levels. This should even have an impact on life expectancy: compared to the general population, vegetarian and vegan people showed lower death rates in several studies on. Of particular note here is the reduced risk of cardiovascular diseases such as heart attacks, the number one cause of death in Austria. In addition, a vegan diet can have a therapeutic effect on various diseases: In rheumatoid arthritis, but also in the case of certain allergies, as well as neurodermatitis and psoriasis, symptoms of the disease can be reduced or even made to disappear completely.

- **Beneficial ingredients**

If you take a closer look at the composition of a balanced vegan diet, the health benefits are not surprising: a diet based on plant foods does not contain cholesterol, less saturated fatty acids and often less total fat, less protein and salt than the usual mixed foods. Instead, it provides people with many essential vitamins, minerals and health-promoting substances such as fiber and secondary plant substances. Of particular note is the significantly higher folic acid content - A vitamin that is mainly found in vegetables and whole grains and is usually not enough in the average mixed food in Austria.

- **Knew how**

Despite these good conditions, a vegan diet is not automatically healthy. After all, it can also consist of finished products, chips, chocolate and cola. As with any other type of diet, a varied diet with a high proportion of vegetables and fruits is important. And like any other type of diet, there are a few special nutrients that should be given a little more attention to avoid a potential deficit.

- **Vegetables and fruits as a basis**

It is well known that vegetables and fruits are the basis of a healthy diet. This applies to an omnivorous diet as well as to a vegan. Implementation is particularly easy with a vegan diet: vegans generally consume significantly more vegetables and fruits than the general population. Here, seasonal, regional organic food should be preferred and the varieties varied. A balanced diet also includes cereal products in the form of whole grains, legumes, nuts and oil seeds, as well as high-quality oils. Here too, variety is the key to a healthy diet.

- **Don't be afraid of protein deficiency**

Protein is found in plant foods abundant: legumes such as beans, lentils, peas and chickpeas, soy products such as tofu, soy milk and yoghurt and seitan from wheat protein, grains, nuts and seeds are good sources. Plant foods contain all essential amino acids. A lack of a varied vegan diet is definitely not to be feared. On the contrary: The somewhat lower protein content even has a positive effect, since too much protein is generally consumed in Austria.

- **Rich in vitamins**

When it comes to vitamin intake, vegans do better than all-eaters with regard to most vitamins. A comparative study by the University of Vienna, Department of Nutritional Sciences, compared the nutrient intake between vegans, vegetarians and omnivores. This showed that the intake of most vitamins and minerals with food was highest in the vegan diet. Only with vitamin B12 and vitamin D were vegans poorly supplied. Because vitamin B12 does not occur in significant amounts in plant-based foods, it should be supplemented in the vegan diet in the form of dietary supplements or fortified toothpaste (available in organic and vegan shops from the Santé brand). Vitamin D can be formed in the skin by sun exposure. It is therefore important to spend a few minutes daily in the midday sun during the summer months. If this is not possible - as well as during the winter months - supplements should be considered.

- **More minerals**

In the study by the University of Vienna, vegans also showed better results with regard to mineral intake. With almost all minerals they achieved a higher absorption - even with iron, which is often mentioned as a potential deficiency nutrient in a vegan diet. However, the iron levels of vegans were somewhat lower despite the higher food intake. This is due to poorer bioavailability of vegetable iron. However, vitamin C can significantly improve the absorption rate. It is therefore advantageous to always eat fresh vegetables or fruit directly with iron-rich foods such as whole grains and legumes - for example, to eat a salad with a lentil stew or a chili sin carne or to drink a glass of freshly squeezed orange juice.

Vegans only showed a poorer intake of minerals with calcium. The calcium requirement can be easily met with plant-based foods, but you should consciously watch out for the daily intake of several servings of calcium-rich foods in order to avoid an increased risk of osteoporosis in old age. Good sources are green vegetables such as kale, savoy cabbage, broccoli and fennel as well as sesame, poppy seeds and almonds, calcium-rich mineral water (from 200 mg calcium / l) and fortified soy milk.

- **The right oils**

The fatty acid pattern is advantageous in principle in a vegan diet, since only a few saturated fatty acids are ingested, which can increase cholesterol levels and favor cardiovascular diseases. Instead, it contains many unsaturated fatty acids that have a positive effect on blood lipid levels. However, you should have an adequate intake of Omega 3 fatty acid be respected. This is contained in linseed oil and linseed, hemp oil and hemp seeds, walnut oil and walnuts, rapeseed oil and chia seeds. A teaspoon of linseed oil or a tablespoon of rapeseed oil cover the daily requirement. However, linseed oil is perishable and should therefore only be used cold and stored in a cool and dark place for only a short time. In order not to negatively influence the conversion to higher-chain Omega 3 fatty acids, the consumption of oils rich in Omega 6 fatty acids such as safflower, sunflower and corn oil should also be restricted. This does not affect oils that have a high proportion of monounsaturated fatty acids and are therefore suitable for heating, such as olive oil or high oleic sunflower oil.

Checklist: vegan nutrition at a glance

- The basis: a varied diet consisting of fresh vegetables, fruits, whole grains, legumes, nuts and seeds as well as high-quality oils.
- Optimize iron intake: Always combine iron-rich foods such as green vegetables, quinoa, amaranth, millet, whole grains, legumes, nuts and oil seeds with vitamin C, i.e. fresh fruit or vegetables.
- Make sure you have enough calcium: Green vegetables such as kale, kale, broccoli and fennel, sesame and poppy seeds, almonds, tofu extracted with calcium chloride, calcium-rich mineral water (> 200 mg / l) and fortified soy milk are good sources.
- Integrate vitamin B12: ideally in the form of supplements and / or toothpaste.
- Spend a lot of time outdoors: plan 5 to 30 minutes a day in the sun, depending on your skin type, during the summer months. Take vitamin D supplements in winter if necessary.

- Choose oils with Omega 3 fatty acids: linseed oil and linseed, hemp oil and hemp seeds, walnut oil and walnuts, rapeseed oil and chia seeds. A teaspoon of linseed oil or a tablespoon of rapeseed oil cover the daily requirement.
- For the iodine supply: occasionally algae, iodized table salt.
- Do not only pay attention to a healthy diet: exercise, moderate to no alcohol consumption and no smoking are important factors that contribute to health.

The essential points of the vegan diet:

- Based on a completely vegetable diet
- Prohibition to consume meat, fish, eggs, dairy products and beehive products
- Need to take a vitamin B12 supplement
- Environmentally friendly and animal welfare diet

The main principles of a balanced vegan diet

The vegan diet goes a little further than the vegetarian diet. Indeed, in addition to meat and fish, it bans the consumption of all products from the exploitation of animals: honey, dairy products, gelatin, etc. In addition to the diet, veganism also very often prohibits the use of animal products in cosmetics and ready-to-wear (wool, leather, etc.).

How does the vegan diet work?

The vegan diet should be balanced and varied. Despite the proscribed foods, the need for different nutrients must be covered by good quality alternative plant foods.

Vegan, vegetarian and vegan: what differences?

These close terms can easily be confused, yet they are indeed 3 distinct typologies:

- Vegetarians consume all food groups excluding meat, fish and seafood.
- Vegans follow a vegan diet which therefore excludes all foods of animal origin (including eggs, dairy products and honey).

- Vegans are vegan and extend this philosophy to many everyday choices: they do not use silk, leather or wool, do not take drugs whose excipients are of animal origin or cosmetics containing ingredients from animal exploitation. Vegans are often vegan, but not always.

The origins of the vegan diet

As early as 1806, there were medical recommendations advising against the consumption of eggs and dairy products. However, it was not until 1948 - with the discovery of vitamin B12 - that veganism became a more widespread diet in society.

How does the vegan diet make you lose weight?

Weight loss is not the goal of the vegan diet. However, cooking vegan requires cooking at home and avoiding all industrial and processed products. In doing so, weight loss is therefore relatively frequent and natural.

How long does the vegan diet last?

Since the vegan diet is more of a lifestyle than a diet, there is no end date. It is a diet often followed throughout life for health, ethical, ecological reasons, etc

Foods allowed in a balanced vegan diet

All plant-based foods will be found on the vegan plate, including vegetables, whole grains, oil seeds and fruits and their derivatives (such as vegetable milks), vegetable oils and fruits.

Foods prohibited in vegan food

In the vegan diet, meats, fish, eggs are to be completely banned. In addition, dairy products, butter, honey and gelatin are prohibited. Indeed, even if the manufacture of these products does not require the killing of the animal it still results from their exploitation.

How a balanced vegan diet keeps you healthy?

Many vegans prefer this diet for health reasons. Indeed, this diet helps prevent certain diseases.

> **Prevention of cardiovascular disease**

With the very frequent consumption of oleaginous fruits rich in monounsaturated and polyunsaturated fatty acids and the absence of animal fats, the cardiovascular system is very well maintained.

> **Limits obesity**

According to numerous studies, the body mass index of people on a vegan diet tends to be lower than the average of the omnivore population since it generally contains less industrial food, and more vegetables and fiber than I omnivorous classic diet.

CHAPTER FIVE

ATKINS DIET

It is one of the best-known low-carb diets and promises quick success on the scales: The Atkins diet. When cardiologist Robert C. Atkins presented his diet plan in the 1970s, he revolutionized all weight loss programs that had existed up to that point. Created by American cardiologist Robert Atkins in the 1970s, the method became known as the protein diet because it prioritizes the intake of this nutrient, in addition to fats, while severely limiting carbohydrate consumption. Animal foods, such as meats (including bacon and sausages), eggs, milk and dairy products become the main characters on the menu. It is also a radical type of ketogenic diet, since it proposes consumption of at least 60% fat and less than 25% carbohydrate in meals - in the traditional food pyramid, these nutrients must represent 30% and 60% of everything that we eat, respectively.

The principles of the Atkins diet

When Atkins published his diet book in the 1970s, his motto was: Fat and protein are allowed, an amount of more than 5g of carbohydrates per day is prohibited during the 14-day initial phase I. He later modified this principle so that carbohydrates are now are also part of the diet in small amounts (up to 20g per day) in the initial phase. The low-carbohydrate diet is supposed to keep blood sugar levels low. Vitamins and minerals should be absorbed through additional preparations. It is essential that, unlike carbohydrates, the body cannot store protein, so excess protein is excreted. This leaves mainly fat for energy production.

There are four different phases in the Atkins diet, which differ in the amount of carbohydrates they consume. People who are very overweight should start with phase 1 in order to get into lipolysis as quickly as possible, especially so-called ketosis, in which the body uses up fat. Phases 2 and 3 mean approaching a higher amount of carbohydrates, but the client continues to lose weight. In phase 4, the client finally eats so many carbohydrates that they neither lose nor gain weight. Atkins saw phase 4 as a lifelong form of nutrition, comparable to today's LOGI method.

- **Phase I (introductory diet)**

Here you should only eat up to 20g of carbohydrates per day for 14 days. According to Atkins, meat offers the optimal combination of amino acids alongside eggs. Soy products can also be used. The permitted amount of carbohydrates should be consumed as a salad and vegetables to avoid constipation. Bread is forbidden. It is recommended that you discuss the Atkins diet with a doctor to check for changes in blood values. Due to the very small amount of carbohydrates, the body is quickly forced to use fat for energy production. The ketone bodies that appear as an intermediate product can be detected in the urine with the help of so-called keto sticks.

- **Phase II (basic weight reduction diet)**

After phase I, nutrition is continued; Now, after the modification of the diet, more nutrient-rich carbohydrates such as vegetables, nuts, berries, seeds as well as beans and legumes can be incorporated into the diet week after week. The amount of carbohydrates consumed daily should be increased by 5g every week, so that in the first week it is increased to 25g, in the second week to 30g, etc.

As soon as you stop losing weight, the amount of carbohydrates should be reduced again by 5g. You now know the maximum amount of carbohydrates you can consume in order to keep losing weight. For most people, the amount should be between 40 and 60g permanently.

- **Phase III (pre-maintenance diet)**

Now the weight loss should almost stagnate. To do this, the amount of carbohydrates can be increased by 10g each week or an additional 20 to 30g of food with a high nutrient density can be added to the diet two days a week, as long as one is still losing weight.

- **Phase IV (lifelong maintenance diet)**

Once the target weight has been reached, the choice of permitted foods increases dramatically: We recommend lots of vegetables, lots of fish and fruit. Pasta and potatoes are still only enjoyed in exceptional cases. Phase 4 is to be understood as a permanent form of nutrition.

What can I eat on the Atkins Diet?

The menu starts with low-carbohydrate foods, e.g. lettuce (lettuce, chicroée, lamb's lettuce, cucumber, rocket, celery) and vegetables (including artichoke, cauliflower, broccoli, kohlrabi, sauerkraut, zucchini, tomato, asparagus, spinach). They are supplemented by high-protein components: Meat (beef, pork, comb, veal, ham), poultry (chicken, turkey, duck, goose), fish (e.g. salmon, tuna, trout, plaice, herring), eggs in any shape (Scrambled eggs, omelets, boiled or fried). Vegetable oils (rapeseed, walnut, soy, grape seed, olive, sunflower or safflower oil), butter or mayonnaise should serve as fat suppliers.

What are the disadvantages?

The absence of carbohydrates and fibers in the initial weeks results in symptoms that may initially discourage those who are not used to dieting: headache, lack of mood and moodiness, nausea, bad breath and constipation mainly. A basic tip to get around the discomfort is to drink plenty of water throughout the diet. It is not recommended to do the diet on your own. The ideal is to be accompanied by a doctor or nutritionist at all times to make adjustments to the menu, if necessary, based on side effects, cholesterol levels (it is important to perform blood tests regularly) and loss of lean and fat mass.

Atkins diet lose weight?

Yes, it is a shock diet, which slims a lot, especially in the first weeks - it is possible to dry up to 8 kg in a month. However, maintaining weight loss is more difficult on this type of diet.

Forbidden food

This diet is based on a carbohydrate restriction, so there are many foods that have no place, at least in its most restrictive phase. You cannot eat cereals, so rice, bread, wheat or rye flours are left out. Also limit the consumption of fruits, especially those that are rich in carbohydrates, such as bananas, apples or oranges. Legumes cannot be consumed for the same reason, during this diet you will not be able to eat lentils, chickpeas, beans or peas. There is no room for starchy foods, such as potatoes. It does not allow the consumption of vegetable oils, except in the case of olive oil, and it prohibits sweets and sugary products. Wow, a near complete restriction of carbohydrates.

What do you base your diet on?

You can eat all kinds of meat, even red meat. Also fish and shellfish, eggs, green leafy vegetables, such as spinach, lettuce, broccoli or chard. Also nuts and, as we have already mentioned before, olive oil. Of course, always raw. It is also important to increase your water consumption to 8 glasses a day, although this is a healthy habit to join our day to day, whether we want to lose weight or not. It also allows coffee and green tea, but all alcoholic beverages are prohibited.

CHAPTER SIX

PALEOLITHIC DIET

In terms of food, the choices must fall on foods that have been the basis for the hunters and gatherers' food - excluding, at the outset, cereals (because the soils in the Paleolithic era were not cultivated) and milk and dairy products (since animals have not yet had been domesticated). Thus, you should choose foods full of nutrients and as natural as possible, that is, that arrive at our tables without or with the least possible industrial processing. Here carbohydrates have no place and fats are eaten sparingly. In fact, this diet has become a success due to the numerous benefits it brings: it helps prevent cardiovascular diseases and diabetes.

It is a diet that is becoming more and more popular within the CrossFit boxes and little by little outside of them as well. But if you still do not know what it consists of, stay that I explain it to you. You hear more and more talk about this diet, although precisely what characterizes it is that it is not a modern diet, based on today if not exactly the opposite. It aims to take us back in time to return to our origins and feed ourselves with what we have been doing for millions of years.

The idea is that in this way, going back to what we have been doing for 2 million years is what our body is supposed to be prepared for. The rationale is that feeding ourselves in this way is the way our body works best, the better it responds, the healthier it is.

History of the Paleo diet

The concept as we know it today we can say that it was born more than 20 years ago. The rationale comes from the so-called Darwinian Medicine, with a scientific publication in the 1991 Quarterly Review of Biology by Drs. George Williams and Randy Neese of the State University of New York at Stony Brook. This publication "The Dawn of Darwinian Medicine" explains how our ancestral past and our evolution affects the way we see and treat disease today. There is a phrase in this study that says that humans are designed to live in stone age conditions. Newer environments can cause various diseases.

What are the advantages of the Paleo diet?

It's time to take care of health. We have to give back to man everything he needs to live healthily. It is time to eat what we want to be. The Paleo diet is the correct solution to change this situation, since it allows to reduce the incidence of chronic and other diseases that appear in an overwhelming way in modern societies. It allows a quick and healthy weight loss, the reduction of blood glucose and insulin levels, and the reduction of risks of heart disease and chronic diseases. Increasingly, the Paleo diet is becoming a diet with enormous healing power. But this diet is not, and cannot be, the same for everyone. Each person has their own specific organic needs and, therefore, must adapt their diet to their physiology.

The Paleo diet is also a way of life:

- In addition to food, we must also respect our genetic essence so that we can prolong life and avoid diseases.

- Measures must be implemented to reduce chronic stress, increase sun exposure and exercise, improve the quality and quantity of sleep.

- Also avoid exposure to chemicals, pollutants, toxics, preservatives and food additives.

- Limit your intake of medications to those that are really needed.

- Supplement yourself, since today's foods do not contain the same concentration of nutrients. Omega 3, probiotics, minerals and group B vitamins and vitamin D are absolutely essential supplements.

What you can eat on the Paleo diet:

- Meat (preferably from animals on Bio pastures and not from animals fed on feed)
- Fish, shellfish, shellfish
- Fresh seasonal fruits and proximity (preferably BIO)
- Fresh seasonal vegetables and proximity (preferably BIO)
- eggs
- Dried fruits and seeds
- Healthy fats (olive oil, coconut oil, macadamia oil)
- Tubers (such as sweet potatoes and yams)

The gray "zone", that is, the foods that arouse controversy among the supporters of Paleolithic food, or that should not be eaten daily, consists of:

- Legumes (Grain, beans, etc.)
- Potatoes and other tubers
- Cocoa
- Wine
- High-fat dairy products (such as butter and ghee).

Some mistakes commonly made in today's Paleo diet:

<u>Variability</u> - In the Paleolithic there was a lot of variety in the diet, however, many of the followers of the Paleo diet have difficulty in varying. It is necessary to vary and introduce different foods daily and respect the origin and time of year.

<u>Way of cooking</u> - the way we cook must respect the temperatures of denaturation of the food. Cooking at low temperatures allows food to keep its nutrients intact and therefore with greater density. We should always include vegetables and vegetables, preferably BIO, and raw.

<u>Ph</u> - The acid / base balance of meals must be respected. To acidifying foods like meat and fish, we must add a generous amount of fresh vegetables, preferably Bio, and raw or steamed.

<u>Fasting</u> - Respect a few hours of fasting or, alternatively, fast 1 day a week.

<u>Salt</u> - The Paleolithic diet was low in sodium and high in potassium, and the potassium concentration the food provided was between 5 and 10 times higher than the sodium concentration. Nowadays, salt is spread and

hidden everywhere and we ingest much more sodium than potassium. On average, the foods that are part of our daily lives provide 3.584 mg of sodium (Na^+) and 2795 mg of potassium, which corresponds to a Na/K ratio of 0.77. For many scientists this is one of the main reasons for the exponential increase in disease today.

Followers of the Paleo diet should therefore eliminate salt consumption and use only fleur de sel, which is rich in all minerals and respects the K / Na ratio. Studies show that changes in this ratio may be the cause of the most common diseases today, such as:

- Initiation and promotion of cancer
- Chronic inflammation
- Deregulation of the innate and adaptive immune system
- Autoimmune diseases
- Cardiovascular diseases due to endothelial syndrome

Sausages, cold cuts and processed meats - Today's sausages and cold cuts, despite being made from meat, do not respect the Paleolithic diet. The way they are prepared, with all the preservatives and salt necessarily used, make them prohibited foods.

Dairy - The human being is the only mammal that consumes milk as an adult and with the aggravating factor of consuming milk of another species. Man only started drinking milk 10,000 years ago, a recent phenomenon considering the history of mankind. The beginning of this consumption coincided with the change from nomadic to sedentary life, that is, when he stopped being a collector and started farming.

However, the human genome has not changed. This is a mutation that takes thousands of years. The profound environmental changes that occurred in the last 10,000 years and that started with agriculture are too recent, on an evolutionary scale, for the human genome to adapt. Milk consumption recently has been associated with cardiovascular diseases, metabolic syndrome, diabetes and osteoporosis. Scientists have identified the mechanism by which cow's milk may also be linked to the initiation and promotion of some types of cancer, such as prostate cancer. It is possible that the same mechanism is behind other cancers that depend on hormone receptors.

<u>**Legumes**</u> - Legumes are foods that are not part of the list advocated by most followers of the Paleo diet. However, there are now some contradictory studies showing that, according to the analysis of the Neanderthal dental plaque, these primitive men ate wild varieties of broad beans and peas, which calls into question the exclusion of legumes from the list of permitted foods. Recently, some researchers like Stephan Guyenet, argue that the Paleolithic man also fed on wild legumes. Legumes have substances considered anti-food, such as lectins and phytic acid (also known as phytate), which makes them potentially harmful.

Lectins are substances that we do not digest and that accumulate in the intestines, which can contribute to inflammation, possible change in permeability (Leaky Gut) and change in immune responses related to Peyer's plaque, which works as a sensor of the immune system in the intestine. The concentration of fermentable substances, FODMAPS (fermentable monc, di and polyols) is probably one of the main reasons why some foods such as legumes, garlic, onions, some fruits and vegetables cause abdominal bloating and gas. However, for most people, the way legumes are cooked can counteract their irritating effect. Soak for about 18 h, cook them in the pressure cooker by changing the water halfway through cooking, or cook them with a little Kombu seaweed are measures that eliminate lectin residues and therefore reduce their action.

These lectins also exist in some fruits, vegetables, spices and other commonly consumed plants, including carrots, courgette, melons, grapes, cherries, raspberries, blackberries, garlic and mushrooms. However, legumes are an excellent source of protein and, sporadically ingested, may contribute to greater food diversity. Many other foods accepted in the Paleolithic diet also have reasonable amounts of lectins, such as mushrooms and some fruits. For these reasons, I am adept at introducing legumes into the Paleo diet, with the following restrictions:

- Maximum 1 time per week
- Only if you don't need to lose weight
- Bake according to the previously explained
- Only if you are not too sensitive and if you do not feel the effect with the recommended cooking method.

Excess meat - If the philosophy is to respect our DNA, then we must also reduce meat consumption. In the Paleolithic man did not eat meat twice a day. Although animal protein is important, excess is dangerous. Meat provides methionine in large quantities, an amino acid that, being very important, in excess can have negative effects on the cardiovascular system. This amino acid is involved in the metabolism of homocysteine, which is synthesized as an intermediate product of the metabolism of methionine by the action of the enzyme methionine adenosyl transferase (MAT). Homocysteine induces direct endothelial damage by producing peroxides that induce changes in endothelial cells and changes in platelet aggregation. If your blood group is not O, then limit red meat to just once a week.

Why does the Paleo diet work?

The Paleolithic diet works because:

- Respects our genetics;

- Eliminates or reduces foods that ignite and cause allergies;

- Controls glucose and insulin levels, reducing peripheral insulin resistance;

- Restores and balances the levels of satiety and hunger;

- It allows good digestion and absorption of food;

- Respects and strengthens the intestinal flora (variety and quantity);

- Highly satiating, allowing a reduction in the number of daily meals.

CHAPTER SEVEN

MEDITERRANEAN DIET

Have you ever imagined a region where people have a high life expectancy and a low incidence of chronic diseases? Because it exists, it is the region bathed by the Mediterranean Sea, which encompasses the south of Spain, the south of France, Italy and Greece. Realizing that these places had so many healthy people, scientists began to study what was different there and came to the Mediterranean diet.

Discovered in the 1950s, this diet has become popular over time. Its main diffuser was the American physician Ancel Keys, who carried out several studies in the region. On the table of the residents of this region is fresh and natural food such as fruits, vegetables, fish, olive oil, oilseeds, grains and cereals. Milk and cheese are consumed sparingly, and wine is also present during meals. Red meat is rarely consumed. Sausages, canned foods and ultra-processed foods are not incluc.ed in the diet. The way they arrive at the table is also part of this way of life. It is part of the tradition of these people to plant, harvest, fish and cook their food, in addition to favoring the purchase of local suppliers and respecting the seasonality of the products. Meals are also always eaten together, as a way to share a moment with others.

Is this diet safe?

The Mediterranean diet is considered safe because it combines not only diversity in food but also a healthier way of life. Anyone diagnosed with celiac disease and lactose restriction needs medical attention to avoid the risk of becoming malnourished, as the dietary pattern recommends both wheat and dairy products. Wine is not mandatory. People with restrictions on alcoholic beverages should remove it from the menu. It is also seen as a good diet for type 2 diabetics. In fact, a study showed that its supporters were 40% less likely to develop this disease than those who did not follow it. It is believed to help insulin work better. The Mediterranean diet promotes the release of the hormone adiponectin, which we all produce, which helps control blood sugar.

Does the diet really lose weight?

The Mediterranean lifestyle is healthier, less stressful and less sedentary. It is linked to the cultural, religious and identity values of a people. Your goal is not weight loss. Choosing this dietary pattern will benefit your health, however, eating large amounts of these foods (even those recommended in the diet) and spending fewer calories can result in extra pounds. If you want to reduce the number of scales, the ideal is to follow up with a health professional. Each has a different caloric requirement. Leaving sedentary lifestyle aside, which these people have been doing for a long time with their daily tasks, can also help lose weight. So, move.

What to eat and drink in the Mediterranean diet

One of the main precepts of the Mediterranean diet is natural food. Processed foods should be avoided, that is, those that have undergone industry changes and that have lost some nutrients and fibers in the procedure. Out of the diet are the sausages, canned and ultra-processed, those products formulated by the industry with little or no fresh food. There are plenty of examples of these products on the supermarket shelves: soft drinks, energy drinks, snacks, stuffed cookies, treats, powdered juice, sausages, frozen products ready to heat, dehydrated products such as instant noodles, powdered soup, cake mix, seasoning ready.

- **Chestnuts and seeds:** almonds, walnuts, macadamia, hazelnuts, cashews, sunflower seeds, pumpkin seeds, and others. They are rich in calories and good fats and help with cardiovascular health.

- **Whole grains:** pasta is a very common food in this region, and it is authorized, but as long as it is whole. Whole grains must replace refined carbohydrates, that is, white flour. Prefer whole products that are a source of fiber, type E and B complex vitamins, minerals such as magnesium, iron, zinc, selenium, manganese, potassium, phosphorus, essential fatty acids, fibers and antioxidants such as flavonoids that contribute to risk reduction for diabetes and cardiovascular disease.

Grains are primarily responsible for providing energy within the Mediterranean diet, but the fact that they are whole gives them a number of benefits. As they do not undergo a refining process, they preserve some important nutrients such as zinc, phosphorus, magnesium and especially their fibers. Therefore, they help to give more satiety, favor chewing and avoid energy spikes that increase hunger and can lead to insulin resistance and subsequently to type 2 diabetes

- **Poultry (turkey, chicken and duck), fish and seafood:** should be consumed at least twice a week. Fish are one of the main components of a healthy diet, many studies indicate the relationship between fish consumption and the prevention of heart disease. Examples: salmon, sardines, trout, tuna. Seafood: shrimp, oysters, crabs, mussels.

- **Low-fat cheeses, milks and yogurts:** white cheeses such as goat and sheep cheeses common in the Mediterranean region can be replaced by Minas cheese, a cheaper option for Brazilians. Yogurts are the most natural (Greek type), with no added sugars or flavors. The most consumed dairy products in the Mediterranean diet are cheeses and natural yogurts, which are the largest sources of calcium in this diet, an important nutrient for bone health. In addition, they are an extra source of protein for food.

Less consumed food

In addition to these mainstay foods in the Mediterranean diet, it also naturally reduces and avoids some types of food:

- **Red meat:** due to a higher intake of fish and also a higher consumption of chicken meat, the Mediterranean diet has less consumption of red meat. People who follow this diet consume only 500 g per week (which is equivalent to between 4 and 5 steaks), which reduces the risk of cardiovascular disease by 11%.

- **Industrialized foods:** The Mediterranean diet has a much higher consumption of natural foods, which reduces the consumption of processed products. This is advantageous since this type of food usually has a high amount of refined sugars, saturated and trans fats and chemical additives that can reduce the quality of life.

What to include with every meal?

Try to add these foods to every major meal: breakfast, lunch, and dinner. If it doesn't work, make up for the deficiency during the day. For example, breakfast without vegetables, and then add them to your snack.

- 125–250g of cooked rice, couscous, pasta and other cereal products or 1–2 pieces of whole grain bread, 40–50g each.

- 150-300 g of fruit. Try to choose different fruits to get all the vitamins you need.

- More than two servings of vegetables 80g each. Choose different vegetables, try to eat at least some raw.

- Olive oil. It is the main source of fat in the diet. Add it to salads, use it when frying.

- 1.5 - 2 liters of clean water, herbal teas on request.

Can vegetarians and vegans eat this diet?

The Mediterranean diet is composed of vegetables, fruits, cereals, seeds, eggs and derivatives, that is, foods present in the daily life of vegetarians. But the diet recommends eating fish and birds at least twice a week. So, to make adaptations and due substitutions, it is always recommended the guidance of a health professional. For vegans, on the other hand, it is a more difficult task, because in addition to meat, eggs and dairy products would be left out of the menu. It is important to individually assess adaptations, but proteins of plant origin can be considered. Examples of vegetable protein sources are: mushrooms, black rice and buckwheat, peanuts, cashews and pine nuts, peas and lentils, and soy tofu.

What can be the menu for the week
I made a menu for a week with five meals: three main meals and two snacks. The diet includes about 1,600 kcal. If you need to consume more or less, choose the serving size yourself.

Day 1

- **Breakfast:** 250 g of spicy apple salad, 40 g of whole grain bread.

- **Snack:** 30g almonds.

- **Lunch:** 100 g of fried salmon fillet with garlic and cherry tomatoes, 200 g of boiled rice, peach.

- **Snack:** 50 g olives.

- **Dinner:** 250 g of pasta with chicken and broccoli in a creamy sauce, 40 g of whole grain bread, an apple.

Day 2

- **Breakfast:** two sandwiches with feta cheese, tomatoes and parsley, an apple.

- **Snack:** 40 g pistachios.

- **Lunch:** 250 g of salad with chickpeas, pepper and feta cheese, 40 g of whole grain bread, pear.

- **Snack:** 50 g of hummus with vegetable slices: cucumber, carrot, bell pepper. Cut vegetables into strips and dip in hummus.

- **Dinner:** 100 g of tuna meatballs, 150 g of boiled potatoes, orange.

Day 3

- **Breakfast**: 250 g salad with spinach, apples, walnuts, cheese and mustard dressing, whole grain bun.

- **Snack:** 150 g ricotta, 20 g walnuts.

- **Lunch:** 250 g of primavera pasta with vegetables, banana.

- **Snack:** 30g almonds.

- **Dinner**: 250 g of couscous with vegetables, 40 g of whole grain bread, a pear.

Day 4

- **Breakfast:** 250g of salad with avocado, grapes, rocket salad, nuts and goat cheese, 40g of whole grain bread.

- **Snack:** 40g pumpkin seeds.

- **Lunch:** 250g pumpkin cream soup, 150g couscous with vegetables, apple.

- **Snack:** 40g olives, 20g hard cheese, cucumber, 2-3 cherry tomatoes.

- **Dinner:** 250g alla putanesca spaghetti, 2 tangerines.

Day 5

- **Breakfast:** 2 whole wheat sandwiches with hummus, apple.

- **Snack:** 5 dates, 30g almonds.

- **Lunch**: 100g of chicken in a creamy cheese sauce with spinach, 200g of rice, a pear.

- **Snack:** 150g Greek yogurt, peach.

- **Dinner**: 250g of Mediterranean herring pasta, orange.

Day 6

- **Breakfast**: 200g spinach frittata, 40g whole grain bread, peach.

- **Snack:** 150g Greek yogurt with a handful of berries.

- **Lunch:** 250g of alla norma pasta, apple.

- **Snack:** 50g of a mixture of nuts and dried fruits.

- **Dinner:** 150g vegetable curry with chickpeas, 150g rice, pear.

Day 7

- **Breakfast:** 250g of apple and honey salad, whole grain bun.

- **Snack:** 150g fat-free cottage cheese with a handful of berries.

- **Lunch:** 250g of fish soup, 150g of vegetable curry with chickpeas, 40g of whole grain bread, orange.

- **Snack:** 30g cashews.

- **Dinner:** 250g of pasta with tomato sauce, banana.

CHAPTER EIGHT

ULTRA-LOW-FAT DIET

The transition to a low fat diet for weight loss is the 70s. New research shows that polyunsaturated and monounsaturated fats promote weight loss, reduce inflammation and reduce hypertension. In fact, the human body needs limited amounts of saturated fat to function properly. Read on to find out if you should follow a low fat diet for weight loss and the benefits and side effects of this diet. However, you can change the numbers and customize your diet plan to suit your health condition as recommended by your doctor. Before moving on to a low fat diet meal plan for weight loss, let's take a look at a few facts about the diet itself.

Basic Conditions for a Low Fat Diet

- Eat only foods that contain 0 grams of fat.

- Do not use cooking fat, such as butter, butter, or margarine.

- To prevent sticking of foods during cooking, use pans with non-stick coating Teflon.

- Add low-fat seasonings (such as ketchup and mustard), spices, herbs, garlic, and onions to flavor your meals.

Do not Eat

Your total daily carb target determines whether you need to limit some of these foods or avoid them altogether. Low-carb diets typically contain 20–100 grams of carbs per day, based on personal tolerance.

- White bread
- Whole-wheat bread
- Flour tortilla
- Bagel (3-inch)
- Banana
- Raisins
- Dates
- Mango, sliced
- Corn
- Potato
- Sweet potato/yam
- Beets, cooked
- Lentils
- Peas
- Black beans
- Pinto beans
- Chickpeas
- Kidney bean

What to Eat on a Low Fat Diet?

Milk products:

- Skimmed milk;

- low fat natural or frozen yoghurts;

- skim cheese;

- other low-fat dairy products, such as low-fat cheeses and low-fat ice cream.

Low-fat or whole foods:

- milk;

- yoghurts;

- puddings;

- cheeses.

Beverages:

- Coffee (black, half-and-half with half and half fat-free product or just with skim milk);

- tea with lemon or skim milk;

- carbonated drinks;

- juices;

- fruit punch;

- low fat hot chocolate.

- coconut milk;

- Cream substitutes;

- cocktails with added dairy products that contain fat (for example, "regular" yogurt, ice cream or milk);

- fruit drinks that should be avoided (see "Fruit" in the "Not to Eat" column).

Bread, cereals and breakfast cereals:

- Porridge or cereal flakes;

- pasta without additives;

- White rice;

- rice noodles;

- low fat white bread;

- Various defatted Muffins Vita and cookies Tops Vita;

- lean rolls;

- matzo;

- crackers Zwieback;

- lean crackers;

- biscuit;

- low fat cookies;

- low fat cakes.

- Any food with added nuts, seeds, or coconut;

- donuts;

- croissants;

- baking;

- pies;

- whole grain products;

- brown rice.

Fruits:

You can eat all fruits, except those listed in the "Do not eat" section, as follows:

- fresh;

- frozen;

- canned;

- prepared in a different way;

- dried;

- jelly;

- jams;

- juices.

- Coconut;

- cherimoya;

- dried figs;

- papaya;

- sapodilla;

- sapote;

- any fruit with a topping containing fat (such as whipped cream).

Vegetables:

You can eat all vegetables, except those listed in the "Do not eat" section, as follows:

- fresh;

- frozen;

- canned;

- prepared in a different way;

- in the form of juice;

- Boca Original Vegan Burger and other vegetarian burgers without fat;

- air popcorn;

- red, black, or pink beans cooked without added fat.

- Any vegetables with the addition:

- butter;

- vegetable oil;

- margarine;

- fat-containing sauces;

- olives;

- chickpeas;

- soya beans;

- avocado;

- canned vegetables with the addition of vegetable oil.

Meat and protein foods:

- Up to 2 servings per day of lean turkey breast or other packaged deli meats marked as low fat;

- egg whites;

- various non-fat Eggbeaters chicken egg substitutes.

- All other products.

A fish:

- All kinds of fish

Fats:

- low-fat butter-like spreads (for example, the Promise and "I Can't Believe It's Not Butter" brands) - up to 2 servings per day;

- medium chain triglyceride oil (available from pharmacies or health food stores) as a dressing for:

- salads with vinegar or lemon juice;

- fruits, for example, for making applesauce;

- frying and sautéing dishes over low heat (not deep-fried).

- Butter;

- margarine;

- all types of oils except medium chain triglyceride oil;

- cooking oil in spray;

- regular salad dressings.

Soups:

- Low-fat broth;

- low-fat soups Health Valley.

- All other products

- Liquid food supplements

- Breeze Boost (Nestlé);

- Carnation Breakfast Essentials vanilla or strawberry flavor powder with added skim milk;

- Ensure Clear (Abbott).

- Ready-to-drink powder or chocolate Breakfast Essentials Carnation;

- any other fatty drinks.

Condiments and more:

- Ketchup;

- fat-free mustard;

- low-fat mayonnaise;

- lean salsa;

- Louisiana "Original" Hot Sauce;

- soy sauce;

- vinegar;

- salted or pickled foods;

- marinades;

- horseradish without additives;

- sauerkraut;

- low-fat salad dressings;

- Molly McButter - up to 2 teaspoons a day;

- low fat pasta sauce;

- pastille (marshmallow).

- regular or low fat mayonnaise;

- nuts;

- seeds;

- olives;

- peanut butter;

- any dishes with added fat.

- MENU EXAMPLES

Double milk

Double milk contains twice as many calories and proteins as skim milk. To prepare double milk and add it to dishes later:

1. Mix 1 liter of skim milk with 1 packet of skimmed milk powder.

2. Shake well and store in the refrigerator.

Example menu No. 1

Breakfast

- Semolina porridge with skim or double milk;

- Boost breeze or ensure clear drink;

- Toast with jelly fried in a dry pan;

- Half and half coffee with half and half or skim milk.

Lunch

- Fat-free black beans garnished with white rice, seasoned with low-fat salsa and low-fat Greek yogurt

- Carnation Breakfast Essentials powder with added skim or double milk;

- Fresh pineapple.

Dinner

- Green salad with low-fat dressing;

- Low fat spaghetti with low fat tomato sauce;

- Green beans cooked in low-fat broth;

- Toasted skim bread seasoned with garlic powder;

- Fruit juice;

- Sponge cake with low-fat frozen yogurt and maple syrup.

Snack

- Fat-free salted pretzels;

- Double milk with skim chocolate syrup.

Example menu No. 2

Breakfast

- Eggbeaters chicken egg substitute with fat-free salsa or ketchup;

- Blue Bran Vita Muffin with strawberry jam;

- Fresh orange;

- Tea with lemon and honey.

Lunch

- Low-fat cottage cheese with fruit;

- Zwieback crackers with apricot jam;

- Strawberry carnation breakfast essentials strawberry flavored powder with skim milk or double milk.

Dinner

- Low-fat veggie burger with ketchup and mustard;

- Baked sweet potatoes with marshmallow;

- Homemade cabbage salad (chopped cabbage, carrots, onions, fat-free mayonnaise and vinegar);

- Fat-free ice cream with fat-free chocolate syrup;

- Fruit juice.

Snack

- Low fat yogurt.

CHAPTER NINE

KETOGENIC DIET

The ketogenic diet is used primarily in the treatment of epilepsy in children. For adults, there is not enough research to support the effectiveness or uselessness of this diet for adults. It is only known that the ketogenic diet is well tolerated by adults and has low side effects. The results of the ketone diet are not proven due to the lack of a control group in most cases. The results can be skewed by the natural disappearance of symptoms. In a little less than half of the cases, children with drug-resistant epilepsy and following a ketogenic diet for more than a year have almost completely recovered from their epileptic seizures. Those who used this diet for only six months received a 90% reduction in epileptic seizures in one third of cases. Studies have shown that dysbiosis is observed in patients with epilepsy, the microbiota in the intestine differs from that in healthy children and adults. In people on a ketogenic diet, the composition of the intestinal microflora improves. Whether the microbiota is associated with epilepsy remains unclear.

The name comes from ketosis, a kind of fat burning induced by the radical cut in carbohydrates. It works like this: by reducing this nutrient, which is the main supplier of glucose that gives energy to the cells, the body seeks other sources of fuel, mainly fat, which is the most ingested nutrient in the ketogenic diet. The process, in addition to using body fat, gives rise to ketone bodies, molecules that interfere with the hormones involved in appetite, such as ghrelin. Ketosis is the main asset of the ketogenic diet, which can vary in shape and ingested calorie limit. In general, carbohydrate consumption is below 50g per day. To get an idea, we usually eat about 200g or more of the nutrient daily.

There is no exact number of meals per day, as each person feels hungry at different times. To induce ketosis, it is necessary for the body to spend time in a shortage of carbohydrates. Therefore, the diet has a minimum duration of 2 to 3 weeks, and can reach 6 months. In general, due to the severe restriction, the program lasts around 40 days. During the first week, which is an adaptation phase, the lack of glucose for the brain can cause side effects such as bad mood, tiredness and weakness. But then the tendency is for the mood to stabilize and the body to "get used" to the new way of making energy.

In the classic ketogenic diet, the consumption of carbohydrates is low (between 4% and 10% of daily calories) that of fats reaches 90% and cannot be less than 60%, and the rest of the calories come from proteins. The amount of calories varies individually, but it is usually between 1000 and 1400 a day. There is also a version that radically reduces the number of calories, to less than 800, the VLCKD (very low calories ketogenic diet) where the number of meals and the menu is more controlled. There are usually six meals ready-made, in powder form, and we only add a few vegetables. Ah, it is worth saying that the ketogenic diet is different from the low carb, which also gained fame for reducing the carbohydrates on the daily menu. In low carb the intake of carbohydrates can reach 150g per day while in ketogenic the limit varies between 20 and 50g.

Foods allowed in the ketogenic diet

The vegetables are all released and most of the vegetables, but several vegetables have to leave the plate, among them potatoes, manioc and the legume family: beans, soy, lentils, peas, etc. The 100% allowed fruits are avocado and coconut, as they are a source of fat. In the field of fats, butter, nuts, olive oil, nuts and lard are also on the menu. In addition to these, meats, fish, chicken, eggs, cheeses, and yogurt complete the list of released. The only drinks that can be drunk are water, coffee and tea without sugar.

Prohibited foods in the ketogenic diet in general, the diet favors natural foods and limits processed products. Here are the items that cannot be consumed:

- Sweets;

- Breads;

- Spaghetti;

- Flours;

- Alcoholic beverages;

- Starches;

- Juices;

- Tubers, such as carrots, potatoes, cassava, yams, etc.;

- Vegetables like corn Legumes, such as beans, soybeans, peas, chickpeas;

- Other sources of sugar cannot be consumed. Attention to physical activities.

Physical exercise must be combined with diet so that weight loss is effective and healthy. However, as the organism is managing itself with little energy, some precautions are necessary. The tip here is to concentrate your carbohydrate consumption before training. For example: a juice containing 100g of watermelon and 100g of beets has approximately 30g of carbohydrates. Now, if you are going to start moving along with the food program, the recommendation is to take it easy. And even if the individual already practices activities, the ideal is to reduce the pace, because some people cannot stand the exercise and may present weakness and cramps.

Is ketogenic diet safe?

First, the diet cannot be done for a long time, as it is very restrictive. Those who have liver or kidney disease cannot follow this diet, as the increase in protein and fat intake can overload these organs. Not to mention that cutting carbohydrates means stop eating various foods with vitamins and minerals important for health, such as cereals, legumes and fruits. Most clinical studies done so far indicate the use of supplements in conjunction with the ketogenic diet. The high consumption of fats is another point to be considered before opting for the plan. Medical societies and international bodies advocate a low-lipid diet. By causing 90% of calories to come from fat, there is a risk of increased triglycerides and cholesterol, which can be a problem for those who already have high levels of these molecules. Because of all these factors, although safe in most cases, the ketogenic diet cannot be done without medical supervision.

Does the diet really lose weight?

Yes. Since carbohydrates make up the majority of meals, cutting them reduces the calories consumed daily which naturally leads to weight loss. Other than that, ketosis consumes body fat, which also leads to the rapid weight loss that made the diet famous.

Is it worth it or not?

The experts heard by the report say that yes, the ketogenic diet has its value, especially in combating obesity and / or metabolic syndrome. Provided, of course, that it is done with monitoring, and has a limited duration of a maximum of six months. There is also a consideration about the menu. For example, there is no point in not eating potatoes but overdoing bacon because it is fat. Finally, the big problem with ketogenic, and with virtually all diets, is keeping the balance hands in place after they finish. It is necessary to find a dietary strategy that makes it possible to maintain the weight lost in the long term.

CHAPTER TEN

PLANT BASED DIET

Plant-based diet means *plant-based diet*. The strategy to dispatch unwanted pounds is a trend in the world. This method does not prevent meat and meat products from being eaten, but suggests that if you are unable to get them off the menu, reduce them with meals. Below are the benefits of this type of regime and how to put it into practice, little by little. If you follow the recommendations correctly, don't worry, the body will not suffer from nutrient deficiency. The plant-based diet, or vegetables, has been widely discussed when it comes to nutrition. Whether due to the positive effects on health, the environment, or the idea of protecting animals, plant-based food arouses people's curiosity. But, after all, does adopting this type of diet mean giving up meat or just adding more vegetables to recipes?

How it works

The idea is to consume most of the natural foods and products derived from plants such as fruits, vegetables, tubers, whole grains, seeds and little animal food, such as meat, chicken, fish, milk and eggs. It is also part of the regime to eliminate processed foods, such as white flour, sugar, oils, margarine, ready-made food and soft drinks. Therefore, it is not a regime focused only on weight loss. "It is a healthy eating habit that preserves the environment", says nutritionist Jéssica Santos.

What foods does the plant-based diet include?

The list of ingredients in plant-based diets is extensive, and some of the most common examples found in Brazilian cuisine are vegetables, such as kale, broccoli, peppers and sweet potatoes; fruits, such as avocado, watermelon, bananas and oranges; pasta and whole grains, such as rice and quinoa; nuts and seeds, such as cashews and flax seeds; in addition to legumes such as beans, peas and lentils. Among the drinks are coffee and teas.

Herbal diet vs. healthy aging

At first, it was discovered during the study that while aging increases the risk of chronic diseases, eating is effective in slowing down this process and sometimes avoiding certain diagnoses. Therefore, the research concluded that the plant-based diet helps to prevent serious diseases that usually develop with advancing age. For example, type 2 diabetes, cancer, as well as cardiovascular disease. Still, they estimated that the risk of suffering from any of these conditions halves. Therefore, eating more plants only benefits the body and the body. In short, this is due to the lower inflammatory potential of the diet. The inflammatory process that the body goes through is called oxidative stress, which is primarily responsible for the development of diseases such as those mentioned. In addition, this methodology is a natural, clean and pure food, which when balanced and well done, provides energy, vitality and adequate nutrition.

How to adhere to the plant-based diet

- Be sure to consult a specialist doctor;
- Start small and make substitutions;
- Gradually include more vegetables in your diet;
- Decrease meat consumption;
- Then, reduce the consumption of other products of animal origin, such as milk and its derivatives;
- If supplementation is needed, talk to your nutritionist.

To start a plant-based diet, it is essential that the intake be varied, including cereals, roots, grains, oilseeds, fruits, vegetables and legumes, always thinking that the more different colors, the more different nutrients will be consumed.

Does this type of diet have disadvantages?

The vegetable-based diet requires attention to the quality of the food that is consumed. Foods such as French fries are of vegetable origin, but they are not healthy and can harm your health when consumed in excess. Another possibility is that discomfort occurs at the beginning of a diet rich in vegetables, until the body gets used to it. This phase can include symptoms such as increased bowel movements, diarrhea or constipation - signs that the body is adapting to the amount of fiber consumed.

CHAPTER ELEVEN

BLOOD TYPE DIET

Created over 20 years ago, the blood type diet suggests that blood characteristics influence the metabolism of certain foods. Thus, each type has a specific menu to have more health, reduce the risk of cardiovascular disease and lose up to 6 kg in a month. The blood type diet is a diet in which individuals eat a specific food according to their blood type and was developed by naturopathic doctor Peter d'Adamo and published in his book "Eat right for your type" which means "Eat right according to your blood type ", published in 1996 in the United States of America.

How the blood type diet works?

Each type has its own book and a very specific menu to follow, with an extensive list of foods that ends up restricting the variety of the diet. Generally speaking, this way:

- Blood type A - Agricultural profile: Without animal protein, based on fruits, vegetables and legumes.
- Blood type B - Nomadic profile: It should avoid wheat, corn, tomatoes, lentils, and increase the consumption of dairy products and eggs.

- Blood type O - Hunter profile: Diet rich in protein and limited in grains and dairy products.

- Type AB blood - Enigma profile: it is a mixture of group A and B. Avoid caffeine and alcohol. Increase your intake of dairy products. grains and seafood.

WHAT TYPE OF MEAL DOES THIS DIET OFFER? EXAMPLE OF A TYPICAL DAY

- **Group O:** breakfast (germinated wheat bread, rice drink, a piece of fruit), lunch (red meat, spinach), dinner (fish-broccoli);

- **Group A:** breakfast (orange, coffee bread), lunch (grated carrots, turkey fillet, tofu, pineapple), dinner (mozzarella tomatoes, olive oil, green salad, pear);

- **Group B:** breakfast (coffee, orange juice, flax seeds), lunch (fillet of herring, carrots, potatoes), dinner (green salad, fried eggs, yogurt, banana);

- **Group AB:** breakfast (tea, spelled bread, strawberries), lunch (tomato salad, lamb chops, green beans, cheese, seasonal fruit), dinner (vegetable soup, sardines, yogurt, fruit).

Benefits of the blood group diet

- It advocates the use of simple, unprocessed foods;
- It can end up getting bored ... because of food restrictions and / or diktats on the lifestyle to follow.

Disadvantages of the blood group diet

- The blood group "diet" does not offer a "diet", by definition transitory, but a lifestyle dictated by the blood group;
- The idea that this diet would be beneficial for health is a matter of belief. They can lead some people to take it long term with:
- A risk of loss of food friendliness and isolation (difficulties in sharing meals with family or friends of different blood groups);
- A health risk linked to long-term food excesses and exclusions (deficiencies, risk of cancer, for example of the colon if the fiber intake is limited and a diet that increases the intake of red meats for a long time);
- A risk of non-compliance with the dietary rules recommended in certain pathologies (for example a renal insufficiency whose blood group

is 0 who would follow the high-protein type O diet would expose himself to a rapid progression of his renal insufficiency).

MYTHS AND TRUTHS ABOUT BLOOD TYPE DIET

1. This type of food works to reduce cardio metabolic risks

Myth. A study published in the scientific journal of The American Society of Nutrition analyzed the ABO genotype, responsible for the blood types we know, and concluded that there is no association between the blood type diet and changes in cardio metabolic disease indicators in overweight adults, suggesting that the theory behind this eating plan cannot yet be considered effective due to the lack of further supporting studies.

2. Blood type A diet may be related to weight loss

Partly true. According to the study released by Plos One, adherence to the Type A diet may be associated with a lower body mass index (BMI), in addition to decreased waist circumference, blood pressure, serum cholesterol, triglycerides and insulin. But this, in fact, is due to the fact that the type A diet is analyzed by the study as the one with the highest consumption of fruits and vegetables and the lowest consumption of meat. Therefore, it is not the blood type that affects health, but the choice of eating habits.

3.   And type O is able to lower triglycerides

Partly true. The same research released in Plos One found that those who opted for the blood type O diet did, in fact, have a decrease in triglycerides in the body. However, as with the type A diet, this is due to the fact that the type O diet is focused on consuming more protein and less carbohydrates, and is not related to each person's blood type.

CHAPTER TWELVE

OVO VEGETARIANS DIET

Vegetarianism is known for its multiple health benefits, including lowering cholesterol. Most of the dishes are made from fruits and vegetables. The vegetarian diet is considerably less caloric and harmful to our body than a current Western diet loaded with processed products. But if it is not well structured it can lead to protein deficiency. The advantage of including the egg in the diet is that it can easily support this possible protein deficiency. Strict vegetarians should take in addition to B12, a vitamin found only in animal products. Ovo-vegetarians can get vitamin B12 from eggs.

Lacto-ovo vegetarians eat everything except dead animals. With this menu you are very close to the current nutritional recommendation for a wholesome mixed diet. This allows only 600 grams of meat and sausage per week, plus two servings of fish. The valuable nutrients that egg, milk and plant eaters miss by not eating meat and fish, easily replace the foods that are still allowed: milk and cheese provide protein, green leafy vegetables contain plenty of iron. And there is also enough vitamin B12 in dairy products. Since children, pregnant women and the elderly have a higher nutritional requirement or poorer nutrient utilization than the average adult, many nutritionists advised them against avoiding meat for a long time.

- Lactovegetarians: as their name suggests, these people consume plant and dairy products (i.e. milk and products derived from milk: yogurt, cheese, butter, etc.).

- Ovo vegetarians: their diet is based on the consumption of vegetables and eggs. This is a very nutrient dense diet that we will discuss in detail below.

- Ovo-lacto-vegetarians: these are people who consume plants, eggs and products derived from milk. Like the previous cases, they refrain from eating meat and fish. It is the variant of the most common vegetarianism in the West.

Different dishes of the ovo-vegetarian diet

We offer you a few dishes that will help you include egg in this type of diet. It will be the ideal accompaniment for dishes based on vegetables, mushrooms and fruits:

- Cooked eggs

- Poached egg

- Carrot pudding

- Scrambled eggs with potatoes

- Eggs with spinach

- Croquettes

- Potato Croquettes

- Dough for noodles

- Creamed potatoes

NOTE

Thank you for reading Diet Express!

Remember, you shouldn't follow the diets listed in this book without consulting your doctor or nutritionist.

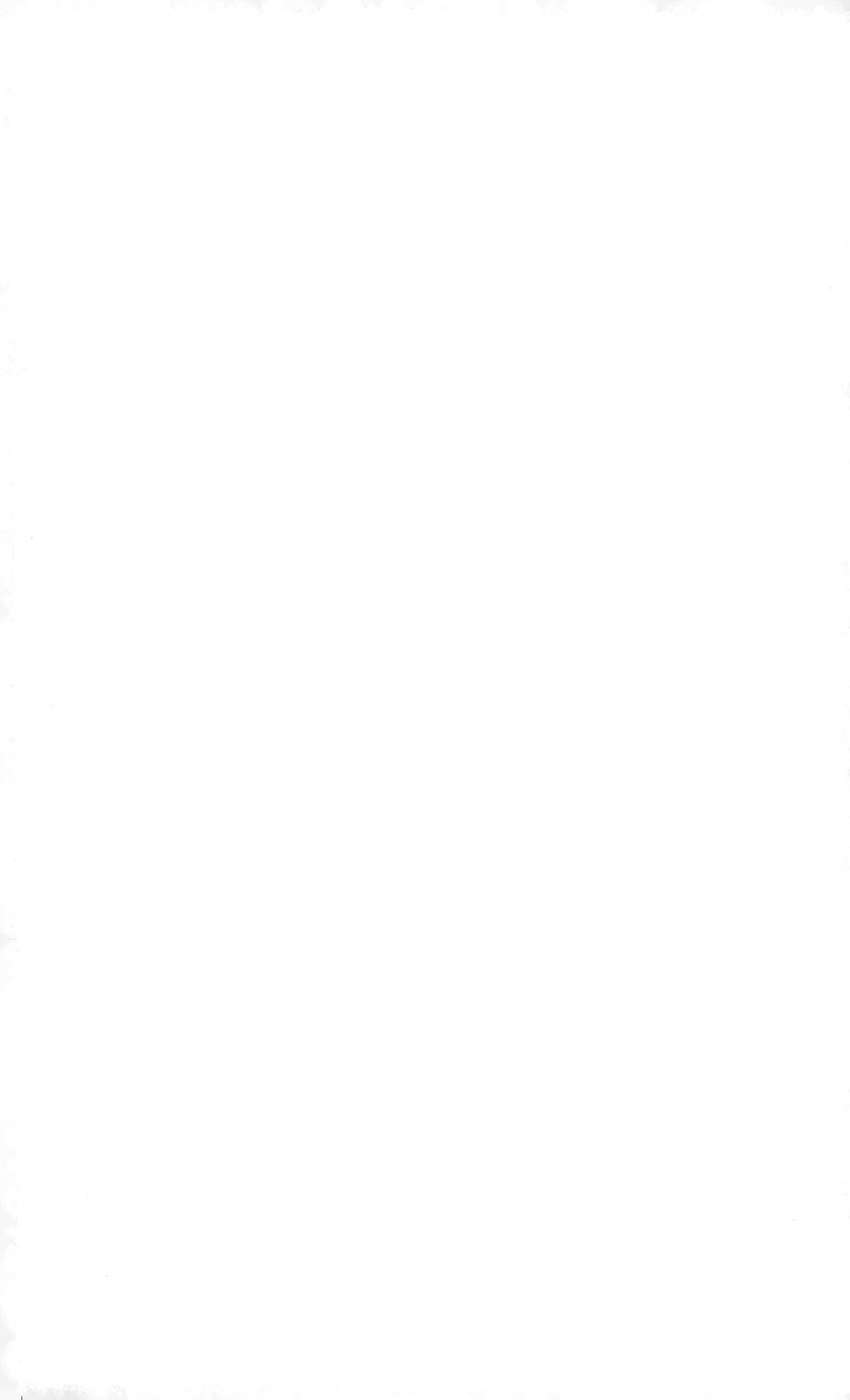

9 798559 363905